FATCOW: FOREVER FIT

By Tracy Kiss

Published by Tracy Kiss at Smashwords

#fatcow My arse wobbles when I walk, my saggy breasts flop onto the top of my podgy stomach to form a little sweat patch when I get hot and my cankles try desperately to break free from the straps of my sandals. I feel horrendous, I'm always tired, paranoid about smelling of body odour and being a single parent means that I can't rest for one moment. I'm a fatcow and I'm going to be single and unloved forever! Something has to change...

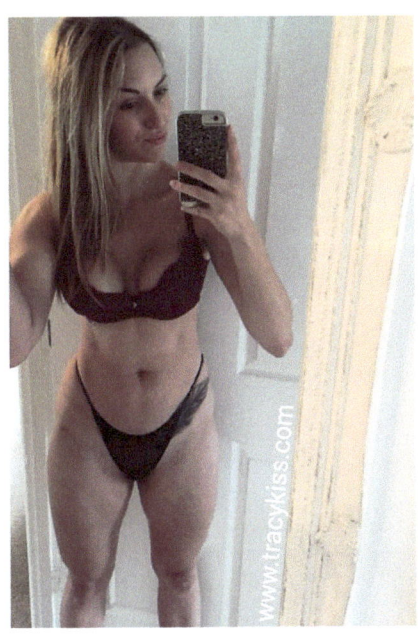

My name is Tracy Kiss, I live in London England, I am twenty-seven years old and this is a selfie I've just taken in my hallway mirror wearing pulled up pants and a mismatching bra as you do! I literally get hundreds of emails and direct messages a day asking me for workout tips and advice from people across the world. But being a single mother to my two children Millisent (7yrs) and Gabriele (3yrs) I sadly don't have the time to be everything to everyone, yet I help charities and strangers as much as humanly possible as I strongly believe in karma and helping to build others up as I build, grow and learn myself. I never sit still for a second and am constantly bouncing from one task to the next just to keep my head above water in my hectic life, and we all know that when time is tight and we're feeling stressed convenience is key, but convenience also makes you lazy, and fat; it's a fact.

Fat seems to have become just as risky a word as racism, sexism and religion, and in this day and age we're so politically correct and keen to not offend that we give offensive words and insults new names to use instead; it's not fat anymore it's plus-size, curvy, real, thick and so on and so forth, but it's all exactly the same thing when you peel back the sugar coating. Whatever way you look at it and whatever you want to call it, being fat is rarely something that we ever aspire to be in life. To some size doesn't matter, but to the majority of the world I would imagine that they feel the same as me when carrying extra weight; unhappy, unattractive and uncomfortable. That's not to say that people of a greater weight aren't beautiful or happy as that's entirely up to the individual and for them to decide how to live their lives. I don't judge others, I just share my fitness journey to motivate and inspire a healthier lifestyle.

So who am I to give advice you might ask? Perhaps I'm a personal trainer, dietician, nutrition advisor or healthcare expert? Sorry to disappoint you but I'm none of the above. I'm just a humble 27yr old mother of two working my way through each day under a mountain of chores and goal posts that always seem to move before I can score. I'm real and what I do to stay in the best shape of my life really works.

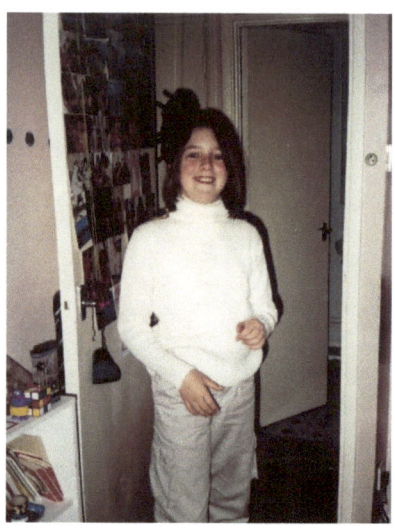

Growing up I've always been the underdog, the quiet, shy little girl who never took part in sports or P.E at school and had no extra curricular hobbies or activities as I much preferred reading a good book to running around with other children at the park. Yet through sharing my lifestyle with the world and my fitness results after having two children I have amassed an incredible following who turn to me for help and advice on achieving the body of their dreams. It costs me nothing to sculpt my body, I visit the gym about as often as I do the dentist and I've maintained my healthy active lifestyle for more than ten years now despite having two children I have never yo-yo'd back and forth with my size. Can I please get a high five for that and now let me show you how to do the same.

Who am I then? I'm not a celebrity, I don't have a personal trainer, flash gym equipment or a personal chef cooking my meals, because let's face it, I'd never have the luxury of such a lifestyle on a single income where my every penny goes to my children. It's just me, myself and I, and occasionally my children hang off of my ankles when I squat or jump on my back when I'm doing press-ups.

Here I'm going to share with you the tips that have gotten me into shape and kept me in shape to this day. What you choose to do with this information is up to you and I must stress that you should always seek medical attention prior to starting a new exercise routine or if you find yourself in pain at any time. Your health is paramount and you need to know your limits.

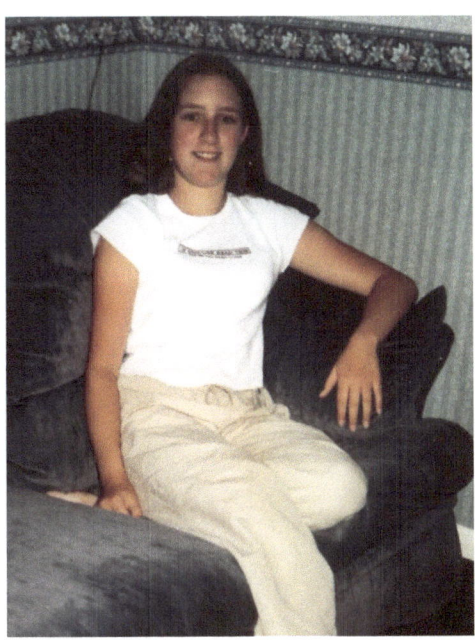

Before you can attempt to change yourself you first need to take a long hard look in the mirror and be honest about what you see. I had my first child at the age of nineteen which was unplanned and I didn't find out that I was expecting until I was already half way through my pregnancy, as it took me passing out and seeking medical help to discover that it was in fact a baby growing inside me that had made me so sick and weak for half a year.

At that time I was very unhappy with my body, I'd been the chubbiest baby ever known to man, with all of the family photos showing plump rosy cheeks and crinkling bands of skin around my wrists and ankles. As I learnt to walk my chubbiness gradually dropped away but I was far from scrawny, I wouldn't class myself as a fat child but I had never been skinny. My tall dad had always loved to keep fit, lifting weights each evening and being my super hero walking around with me on his shoulders. On the other hand my short and petite mum was as strong as an ant, had enviable biceps and was always on the go. As the years have ticked past my dad now sports a middle age spread and my mother is frail, I guess it's the effect of age and time, but what I'm trying to say is that my family are fairly average people, hands on and healthy and of my cousins, aunts and uncles none of us are skinny. So I can't play the good-genes card here and say that I'm in great shape because my family are all perfectly slim supermodels, nor that I've been out of shape because my family are obese, we're just average. If we eat too much we get fat, if we cut back we lose a little chub.

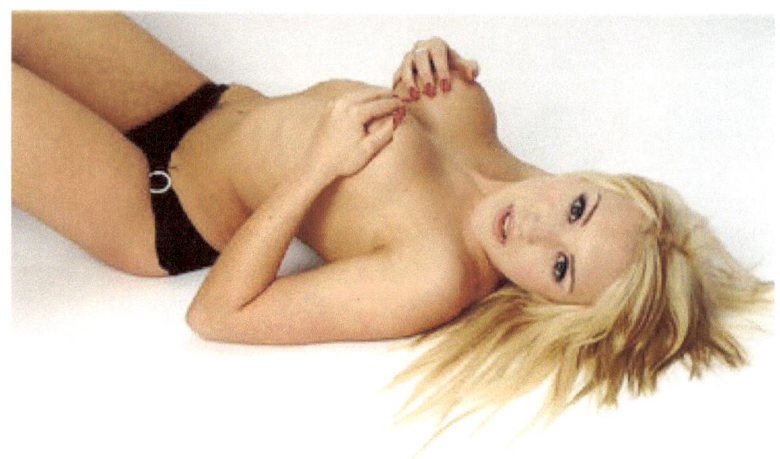

Anyway, back to my pregnancy. At the time I was a model and I was ridiculously neglectful to my body by limiting my intake of food to the point of severe hunger, ironically I didn't like anything about myself yet others constantly praised me about my perfect body. I was convinced I was too fat despite my hipbones and ribs sticking out and when I looked in the mirror at my perfect skin and enviably toned stomach all I saw were faults and flaws. Being around other models didn't help, as it was a catty and competitive environment and battle of the wills over who could be the skinniest. I remember sitting next to a girl on a photo shoot and hearing the loudest stomach rumble that just wouldn't stop, we looked at each other accusingly but didn't know which one of us it was, in hindsight it was probably both. I would drink cups of boiled water to stave off hunger and some days I'd only have a single banana or carrot, convincing myself the hunger pains meant that it was working because the other girls did exactly the same. Eventually my periods stopped for a few years and my doctor warned me that I was underweight and wasn't healthy, but as I was never diagnosed as anorexic I never received any help or support for how I felt and treated myself.

Personally I think that my hatred towards my body as a young adult stemmed from being bullied throughout school for being 'ugly', I felt worthless and wanted to change everything about myself. But maybe it's something that we all go through in life at one point or another, self-doubt, disgust and unhappiness with our appearance. Either way it's unhealthy and stupid as hell so don't even go there!

With no periods for years I had no sign that my contraceptive pill had failed, I was always tired anyway from not eating properly, had stomach cramps from hunger and had to be given suppositories by the doctor to help me to empty my bowels because my insides were dehydrated from my lack of fluid. I only ever drank water when I absolutely had to but even the smallest amount would make my stomach churn, leaving me feeling like I'd swallowed an ocean that slopped around inside of me and only made the hunger feel more painful. I've hardly ever felt thirsty in my life, it seems to be a reflex that I just don't have, and because I never drank I had frequent water infections from the strong toxins building up in my body, it hurt so badly to go to the toilet that I needed medical help and I detested my body all the more for it. How unglamourous forced skinniness is.

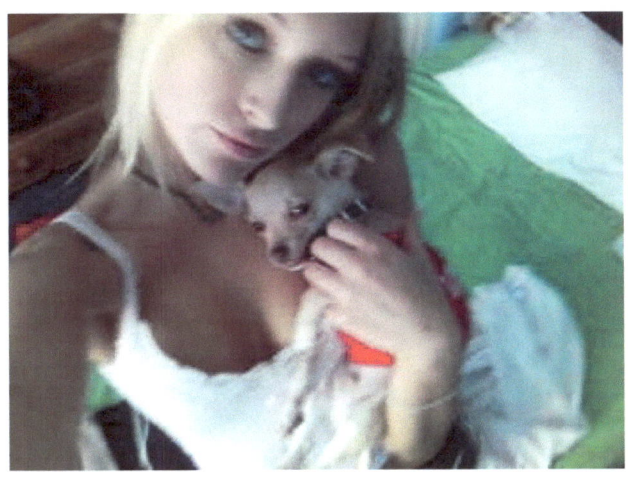

So it's safe to say that my own body pains and problems at the time had managed to mask the symptoms of pregnancy. Being stupidly skinny meant that I never had breasts, so I paid for my own cosmetic surgery when I was eighteen to have silicone implants from a 30A to 30DD which grew almost several sizes whilst I was pregnant, but I put it down to my natural breasts finally developing and never thought in a million years that there was a baby hiding away inside of me as my stomach remained exactly the same, tight and flat as a pancake.

I still remember the shock and sickness I felt when I was told that I was pregnant, I was sitting down after fainting and my head wouldn't stop spinning, my heart beat so hard and loud that it felt like it was in my ear. As a young naïve teen I couldn't accept it, I didn't want to believe it and I certainly didn't want a baby because I wasn't ready to grow up or be responsible. It felt like the end of the world and I just wanted to bury my head in the sand and make everything go away. At the time I was single and almost half way into my pregnancy, calling the father he told me he was too young to be a dad and didn't want anything to do with us, so I was entirely on my own and petrified. Seeing my daughter for the first time on the ultra scan fully formed and sleeping peacefully inside of me thankfully gave me the wake up call that I needed and my life changed enormously that day which I shall forever be grateful for.

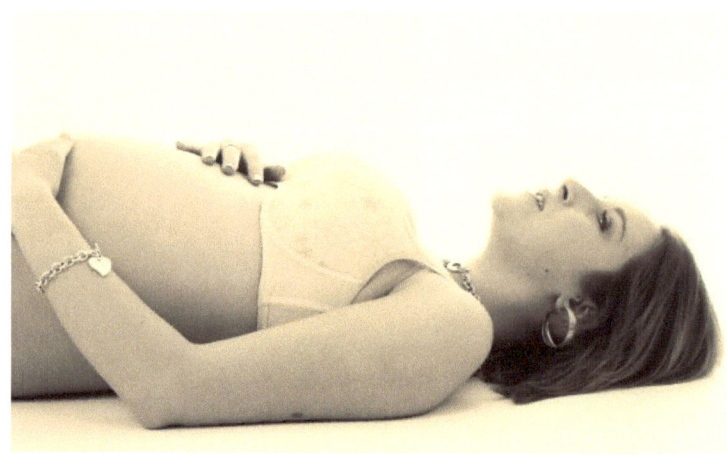

With the knowledge of a tiny life growing inside of me I stopped thinking about myself and my body and thought only of her, switching my on/off starvation for full-sized meals with my relieved family and any food that I craved or desired. Pregnancy introduced me to my love of food, where I had always denied myself calories I went on to eat myself silly with literally anything I could get my hands on. It started out that food made me feel better, it took away the hunger pains and gave me the energy to remain awake, but then I discovered sugar, sweets and treats and I craved it all, not just because of pregnancy but the excitement over having everything I had always forbid myself. I went from having total control over my body to no control at all, and I justified it to myself at the time that I was eating for my daughter to make sure she was healthy, although perhaps rice pudding, ice cream, semolina, ginger nut biscuits and spinach and ricotta baguettes weren't the healthiest of pregnancy foods, but I really enjoyed eating and I'd never even tasted such foods before. I happily drank five pints of full fat milk each day after always refusing it as a child when I became a vegetarian at the age of five, the first person in my entire family to deny meat, and then suddenly craved dairy products during my pregnancy, which may have been down to the fact that I had weak bones and a lack of calcium and iron.

Some people can eat anything they like and stay slim and the other 99.9% of humans have to work hard at it. I'm sadly not in that 0.01% and that's probably not a shock to you either. So my pregnancy eating didn't just make my baby grow but it also made me grow, and rather than gradually putting on weight throughout my pregnancy it seemed that within just a few short weeks of discovering I was in my second trimester I went from ill-looking to gigantic as my body ballooned and revelled in the new experience of being fed. At 38wks into my pregnancy I was so huge that I found it hard to breathe with my daughter sitting high up under my ribs, my breasts were massive and my bras dug into my shoulders, my belly stuck out so far that I couldn't see my toes, my ankles were constantly swollen so I lived in flip-flops and I had awful back ache and heartburn. Everything about me felt pumped-up, inflated, hot, heavy and a chore to move my body but I loved being pregnant, I bloomed with happiness and loved finally being allowed to eat as well as being incredibly excited to become a Mummy. When I stopped worrying about trying to be perfect I actually started enjoying myself and I fully understand how eating makes people happy but quickly gets out of control.

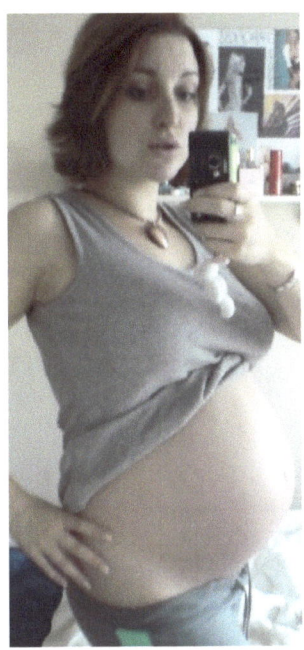

But then my skin tore because the pressure on my body from my dramatic weight increase was so tight that it tingled and burned, and one morning when I woke up I looked down to see hundreds of dark red scratches dug into my skin all over my stomach, hips and thighs. It was as if a cat had scratched and clawed at me in my sleep and I thought that I was covered in blood because I'd never seen anything like it before. My skin had been pushed to breaking point and gave up the fight, I was now the not-so-proud owner of a body tainted by stretch marks, fat and wheezing as I tried to roll up out of bed to plod over to the mirror to assess the damage; yet all that I could see were the dark red cuts all across the front of my stomach and hips as my large bump hid my thighs and lower belly. I cried my eyes out at what I'd become and my insecurities and low self-esteem were by far the worst they've ever been right then, I mourned the skinny body I'd had just months before and hated the disgusting disfigured mess I'd become. Just seven days later I gave birth, becoming a single parent to my 39wks healthy happy 7lb daughter Millisent Kiss, who was my angel Millie-Sent-From-Heaven to save me. And I truly owe my life to her.

Giving birth wasn't fun at all and I'm glad that I knew nothing about what I had to go through beforehand because I would have panicked all the more if I'd have know. Sometimes ignorance is bliss in life, and I'm forever thankful that my mother held my hand and wiped away my tears to get me through it because the moment I first held my daughter all of the pain and hurt instantly went away and I felt nothing but love.

Ridiculously I expected to be skinny after giving birth because surely my baby was out and I could be me again, nuh-uh! It turns out that I wasn't actually expecting quads for the great size of me, just one average sized baby and the rest was solid body fat, eek! Being a young working single-parent I was tested to my limits when raising my daughter alone, breastfeeding until my nipples bled, up all night rocking her desperately in my arms to stop her from crying, and falling asleep standing up as I rinsed out the blender to make up some more organic homemade baby puree. I became a robot living on next to no sleep, my eyes constantly burning and stomach churning from tiredness as dark circles crept out from under my eyes, my hair thinning and my skin pale. Looking back I don't know how I managed it as such an irresponsible teenager, I had nobody to do it for me so unwittingly I learnt how to do it all by jumping straight in at the deep end and it made me the confident and capable person that I am today.

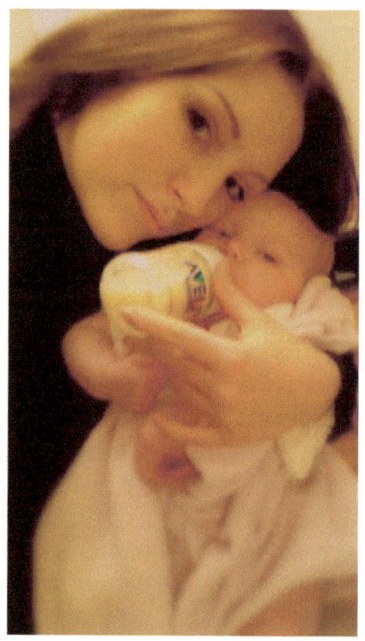

I took to motherhood like a duck to water, busying myself with my daughters needs rather than my own. I still had such an amazing love of food but my home cooked meals for myself would sit on the kitchen table going cold as I stopped to breastfeed, change a nappy or do the laundry first whilst she napped. I found myself forever running around from one task to the next, working night shifts in a bar whilst she slept and studying for a diploma from home during the day between cuddles and feeds. My greed towards food could have easily continued after giving birth if only I had the time to actually stop and eat, and whilst I no longer stuffed myself silly I never went back to starving myself either. I just ate as and when I could remember to, grabbing whatever was available and cooking as quickly as possible before leaving for work and midwife check-up appointments.

Yet when I looked at my reflection in the mirror, my stretch marked crinkled saggy stomach hanging over my jeans, my heaving breasts sitting inches lower than before and my thinning hair and fraught nerves I realised that it was time to look after myself as well as my daughter. I'd put on almost four stones in weight during my pregnancy and had well over two stone still left to shift after her Christening. I lived in baggy clothes, the classic Mum-attire, jeans, trainers and a shapeless t-shirt to skim over my lumps and bumps, pulling on a woolly jumper if I got chilly or donning a kaftan in the sun; anything to ignore and hide away my body.

But hiding what you hate won't ever get rid of it, running away from your problems won't ever fix them, it's just a distraction and they will wait mockingly for you, constantly reminding you of your insecurities and failures everyday when you reluctantly take your clothes off at night and get dressed first thing in the morning. Raising a child as a young single parent is ridiculously hard, but I loved it warts and all, I loved my daughter more than anything in the world and I wanted to make her proud of me, to be able to run around at the park together and feel comfortable in a swimsuit to take her on holiday and smile in pictures instead of running away from the family photo album feeling fat and disgusting.

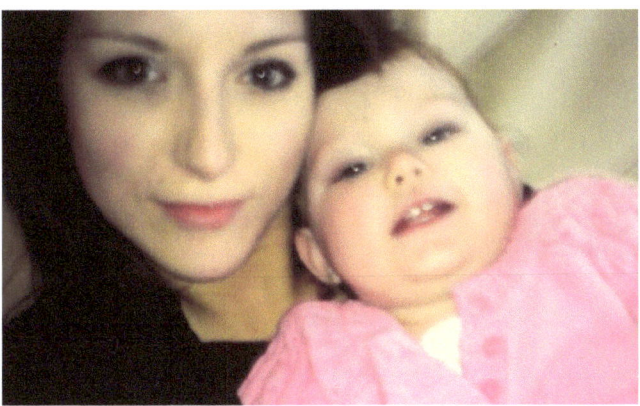

So something had to give and the first question that I asked myself was *why am I fat?* That's easy right, I'm fat because I've had a baby and it happens to every woman, my body changed with pregnancy and I put on weight; um, no! I put on weight because I ate to excess, pregnancy doesn't equal fat it equals a baby. But it's not a bad thing putting on weight during pregnancy, God knows that us girls have a hard time of it, our hormones are all over the place, our bodies are changing beyond recognition and it scares us, we feel ugly and unkempt and comfort eat along with the most uncontrollable cravings for bizarre food at all hours of the day and night. So don't be so hard on yourself if you pack on the pounds when you're expecting, it's a time when you can totally get away with it, have a little fun with food and let yourself go if you need to, just be prepared to work your arse off, literally, after it's done in order to reclaim your body.

Whilst I don't condone unhealthy eating during pregnancy, we all have things that make us happy in life, things that bring us comfort and calm our nerves at stressful times, so have every food group in moderation is more sensible as you should never put yourself or unborn child at risk. It's bad enough damaging your own health, but your baby could be allergic or harmed by food contracting poisoning so avoid mould-ripened cheeses, unpasteurised milk and soft cheeses, raw or runny eggs, liver, cured meats, raw fish, caffeine, alcohol, tobacco and drugs. If you really want chocolate have a cube instead of a bar, if you desperately need ice cream have a scoop instead of a bowl or better still make your own from healthier ingredients and home-grown vitamin rich fruits and vegetables.

Ok, so I'm not fat because of pregnancy, I'm fat because I lost my self control and overate, yet when I had self control I used it in the wrong way to starve and punish myself and that wasn't a great idea either. I've seen both sides of the coin and worn the crown for each, the skinny bitch vs. the fat cow, and I don't want to be either of them because they both suck. But that still isn't the reason why I'm fat, so I questioned why I starved myself with self-control and realised that it was because I didn't like the way that I looked. And why didn't I like the way that I looked? Because I'd always been bullied for being ugly growing up. Other children had hurt me for so long that even after I'd escaped them by leaving school I still continued to hurt and punish myself because I was so used to it.

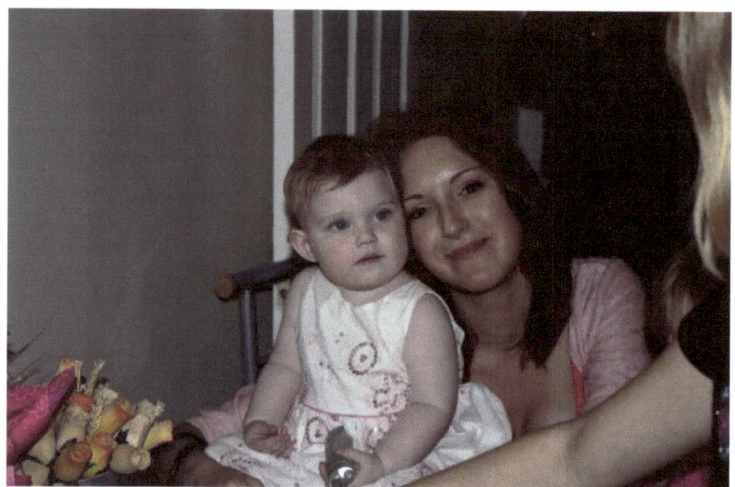

Despite being deemed as beautiful as a blonde leggy model, I hurt myself by denying myself food. I felt worthless and angry at how I was treated, and in turn I treated myself badly. I changed everything about my natural self, used sunbeds to darken my skin, dyed my hair peroxide blonde, had nail extensions, hair extensions, contact lenses and wore head-turning outrageous outfits, a million miles away from the shy quiet girl that I was growing up, I used beauty to mask my insecurity but it was all false and I still hurt inside.

Now that I'd found my reason for being fat, because I didn't like my natural appearance, I needed to fix the problem before I could look at transforming my body, as much like driving a car on flat tyres you can cover the puncture with reels and reels of sellotape and glue but eventually it's going to let air out again and damage the wheel until it's damaged beyond repair. And although it may seem like a big and expensive job to buy four brand new tyres for a car they'll last far longer and actually get you to where you're going safely and on time. Instead of running away from something, papering over the cracks or making-do with tools unfit for the job, face your issues head on and deal with them once and for all and then you can get onto the task of earning the body of your dreams.

We all have our underlying issues in life that cause us to overeat, perhaps it's from feeling unloved, unappreciated, over worked, under paid, unattractive or worrying about bills, responsibilities and an uncertain future. There's no doubt about it, in times of need our hunger goes into overdrive and whilst a bar of chocolate and whole pack of cookies may feel like a distracting haven at the time we're smashing our gums through them, they always make us feel like absolute shit after the crumbs settle and we realise how greedy and reckless we've been.

So take an unhappy relationship and talk to your partner about how you truly feel, put your emotions, concerns and hopes out there vocally and lay your cards on the table, fix the relationship if it can be fixed or cut your losses and walk away whilst you still can. Don't live in a hellhole of a depressing ground-hog day for the rest of your life just because you're afraid of change or being on your own, it's far more painful remaining with the wrong person in life than it is to go at it alone and actually be happy as an individual. Change is beautiful and it will happen for the rest of your life whether you like it or not, so embrace it now and own it before it owns you and life will be so much better.

If you feel trapped at work and underpaid then ask yourself if you're making the most of your career, do you still want to be at the same job you're in now for another five years? If the answer is no then hand in your notice and go do something you actually enjoy, you're going to be working until the end of time anyway and forever is too long to constantly do something you despise. If you love your job but don't feel appreciated then speak to your boss, tell them your talents aren't being fully utilised and be bold, stick your neck on the line and ask for more responsibility, prove your worth and test your limits. You never know you may just get a promotion, a personal assistant, your own office or company car for thinking outside of the box, get one step up on the ladder and make a worthwhile contribution and you'll love the satisfaction and perks that it brings.

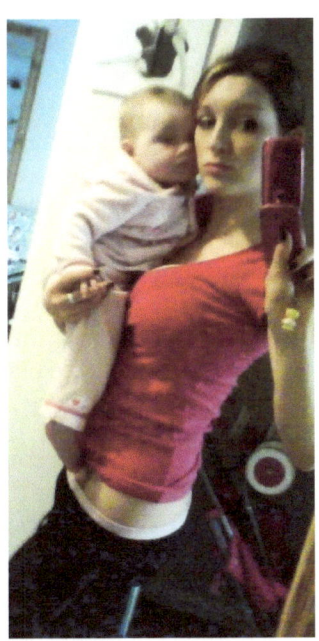

If you stress about money and have no way to make more then start from the bottom up and look at what you're spending your earnings on each month. Make a list of everything that comes in and everything that goes out and decide what is necessary and what's a luxury. Do you really need to have the latest phone, trainers and bad habits or expensive hobbies? Could you switch to a pay as you go simcard instead of contract? Trade designer labels for wardrobe staples, buy non-descript plain clothes that you can wear with anything, if a fashion-branded t-shirt normally costs you £35.00 then a plain black one from a supermarket might only cost you £4.00; snobbery doesn't pay the bills and nobody can see the label when you're wearing it anyway. If a gym membership is crippling you then get some second-hand basic equipment to workout from home, car boot sales are always full of bargains. If rounds of golf, football games, shopping trips and nights out leave you overdrawn then cut back on them and instead wait until you've saved enough money first before going on a night out rather than spending it before you've earned it. If you absolutely have to go out drinking then buy some bottles of alcohol from the supermarket and have a few pre-drinks at home with some friends first, it'll cost half the price of drinking in a bar and you'll only need to buy a couple of drinks when you're out to get drunk rather than several rounds if you go out sober. Whatever clothes you haven't worn or gadgets you haven't used it in the past year go and stick them up for auction on eBay or at a car boot sale, not only will you have more cash in your pocket but your home will be cleaner and clearer and the stuff you do love and actually use can be stored more safely. Clear the clutter and fill up that wallet.

It's amazing how quickly spending can amount to waste over days, weeks and months of unnecessary and greedy behaviour. As a single parent I have to watch my pennies just as closely as I watch my children when we hold hands to cross the road each day. When you become conscious of your spending you will start making better informed decisions when out and before you know it you could save a few hundred pounds each month which would be the equivalent to a raise in wages, just for being spending savvy. Take for example the fact that my children are literally obsessed with Hula Hoops, you know those salted potato rings that you can poke on your fingers before you eat them, they come in a tiny bag perfect for snacking and school lunch boxes, devilishly convenient and such wasted calories. Well the kid's love them but I refuse to stock my kitchen cupboards with them because crisps are unhealthy, unnecessary and a waste of the weekly shopping budget. My local supermarket sells a large 7xHula Hoops pack for £1.75 which is a weeks worth of crisps for one child right? But children like to be treated equally and it's tantrum central if they don't have exactly the same each; so I'd need 14 packs of Hula Hoops each week to give them just one tiny 24g bag a day, which is practically all air as it amounts to a couple of handfuls of finger crunching if you will to the tune of £3.50 a week, £14.00 a month and £168.00 a year, for a snack! Unnecessary junk food at its finest.

£3.50 a week at Aldi where I do my food shopping could provide a ridiculous amount of food for our dinner table. Aldi do a weekly Super 6 where they take six random fresh foods and sell them for £0.39p each and after a quick search on their website just now I can see that they're currently offering: a 6 pack of salad tomatoes for 39p, a cauliflower for 39p, a 500g pack of chantenay carrots for 39p, red and white cabbages for 39p each, a 1kg pack of white onions for 39p and 179g of white and red grapes for 39p, the entire amount totalling £2.34, that's saving me £1.16 on the cost of a quick snack once a day for the kids and filling my fridge with fresh and nutritious ingredients rather than artery clogging fat. Already my mind is ticking over what meals I could prepare from that, perhaps I'd use the cauliflower, carrots and cabbage to put with some roast onions and potatoes for Sunday dinner, the tomatoes to slice onto rye crackers for a light lunch and the grapes as a healthy incentive to encourage the children to walk to and from school or for a nice treat after finishing their dinner in place of a cake or pudding.

So just from taking away the unnecessary snack of Hula Hoops from my weekly shop I can cover the majority of the weekly food shop for a family of three, all I'd need is a loaf of bread for school lunches, 4-pints of fresh milk for the morning cereal, some fruit and potatoes as I'm now vegan and the children and I eat soya that I have stocked up in my freezer because it's low in fat and a great source of protein, a perfect meat-free alternative for all diets.

Take this snack example and apply it to the rest of your daily routine, perhaps a daily pack of chewing gum, newspaper, cup of coffee from the vending machine or meal deal at the newsagents on your lunch break eats into your weekly wallet. Spending an unnecessary pound each day on treats is still £365.00 a year and I just got my annual comprehensive car insurance policy for £299.00 by paying it outright at my renewal. What's more important, car insurance or chewing gum? It's not about being tight or a Scrooge, but savvy with your spending and recognising what is a luxury and what is a necessity, a necessity will keep you alive and a luxury will make you broke and fat. Smoking is a luxury, and a dirty one that that, it costs several pounds a day to buy a single packet of cigarettes which is a ridiculous £2,500 a year; as well as increasing your chances of heart disease, having a stroke, cancer, pulmonary disease and the daily joys of headaches, nausea, fatigue, difficulty concentrating, depression and insomnia to name but a few. So ditch the fags and improve your health, stick half of the money you've saved into the bank for a rainy day, clear off some debts, go on holiday and spend some quality time with your loved ones and you'd still have change left over for a personal trainer and annual gym membership!

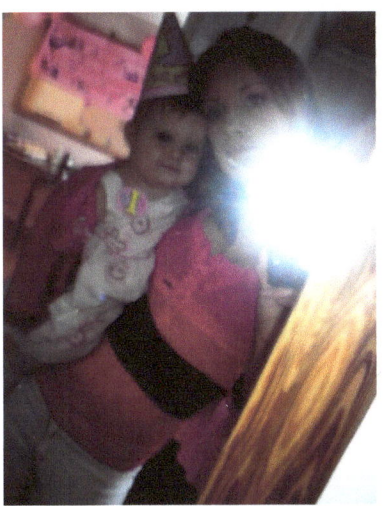

Ok, so that's your love life, job and money problems sorted, yes it really is that easy once you start making changes, stay patient and consistent and watch your problems dissolve before your eyes. Now let's sort my problem, feeling disgusted by my body, or my body dysmorphic disorder if you will. Yes I starved myself, yes I've had surgery in order to feel attractive and complete and yes I wanted to have control over my appearance, weight and life by being obsessively compulsive, but where did any of it get me, deathly skinny and now ridiculously fat after giving birth. The sad fact is that we will very rarely love our appearance or be happy with the reflection that we see staring back at us in the mirror. We're surrounded by celebrities, film stars and models glistening from our television screens and pouting from within glossy magazines and in comparison we feel like we are ugly trolls, but we're not, they just don't live in the real world. Take it from me and my days as a model, those *perfect* girls were always moody, snappy, hungry, tired and shallow as would anyone be when they obsess over their appearance, starve and deny themselves on a daily basis just to please others. You really wouldn't want to be them, ever.

So when I became a mum I was pretty tired constantly, I had very little time to myself, became surprisingly forgetful from messing up my sleep pattern, my diet was all over the place and my body looked horrendous to the point that I couldn't look in a mirror. I looked like a saggy deflated balloon only I still needed to finish deflating in order to be slim again, my skin was loose, stuffed with fat and flabby and I'm now covered in stretch marks, my skin is dry, my hair thin wispy and all of my nails weak, chipped and broken. I breastfed my daughter for a few months before my milk blocked up from mastitis and I lived on cold dinners and nibbles throughout the day. I ate as and when I remembered that I was still conscious, before collapsing onto my bed face down in the early hours of the morning only to be woken up by incessant crying from my daughters trapped wind and smelly nappies that resembled the fragrance of rotting road kill.

I didn't love myself, I didn't like myself and I couldn't stand looking at my body in the mirror, in fact even putting on makeup in the bathroom cabinet at head height pissed me off because of my double chin and lack of any jaw line or cheekbones. I was a pale plump mess and also a single parent. So let's bite the bullet and acknowledge the cards that I'm holding here, there's not one thing that I liked about myself so the only way was up right? I'll never get rid of my stretch marks, I'll never have my perfect pre-pregnancy body back but when I had it I didn't appreciate it anyway, so what have I actually lost? Nothing really, if anything I was visually worse off for being fat, and most importantly not wanting to be fat, but I was still me and far stronger as an individual for what I'd been through and I wouldn't change my daughter for the entire world despite what pregnancy did to my body. If you feel sorry for yourself and play the victim then life will shit all over you, you'll get left behind, downtrodden and become an easy target. It's fine to cry, to feel bad and feel useless, but after you're done with the puffy eyes and blocked up nose pouring your heart out then suck it up, man up and find the guts to actually do something about it and change yourself. I realised I had to change my lifestyle to sort myself out, and although I couldn't erase my scars I just had to accept them because even men get stretch marks and it wasn't like anyone was going to see me naked anytime soon anyway. I'm human, in a world filled with fellow humans and nobody is perfect. Recognising my flaws, facing them head on and knowing in my heart that I don't want to be this size anymore was the first step on my road to recovery. Some people have the wake up call straight away, others can take years to realise that they can't take anymore, regardless of how long it takes you to want to change, just knowing that you're ready is the biggest step of all.

Now I'm not going to tell you to give birth and get your arse straight to the gym, nor if you're heavily overweight to go and do hours and hours of crazy exercise, as it has surprisingly very little to do with the grand scheme of keeping fit compared to your diet. For men reading this or women who don't yet have children, you don't have to have a specific reason or cause for being fat, you just have to want to change. Changing isn't a chore or to-do list that you can bullet point, it isn't to please your partner or to make others like you more, it's something that you actually want to do for yourself and absolutely nobody in the world can do it for you. There is no quick fix, no magic wand or easy way out, but there are baby steps that you can take that will soon become giant leaps for mankind over the course of nine months and my two children are proof of that.

So sort your shit out before you even think about dropping your dress sizes, because no matter how hard you try or how much you think that you want something, if the problem causing your weight gain in the first place is still there then you will never succeed until you remove the fuel from the fire. Start today and face your problems head on, your weight isn't your problem, the reason you gained it in the first place is, and more often than not it's because of bullying, work, love or money. When you remove the stresses from your life you're not as pushed to want to comfort eat or binge and you can build a stronger more reliable foundation that will keep you consistent and on track. Look to change your lifestyle not just plan to be healthy for the next couple of weeks because that's how yo-yo dieting happens and we actually want to stay fit and trim for life, just as I have done.

I don't believe in dieting because it's all really just a fad, whether it's drinking soups all day or only eating chicken, your body needs energy, it needs vitamins and minerals and nutrients to function properly and you can't get that from limiting your calories to nothing. I've told you why starving is an horrendous idea and so dangerous for you, and I hope now that you can understand what has caused you to get to this point in your life. I do not want you to punish yourself; I do not want you to hate yourself, feel sad for yourself or incapable. I want you to hold your head high take a deep breath for me and know that I am here for you every step of the way because I believe in you. I did it and you will too.

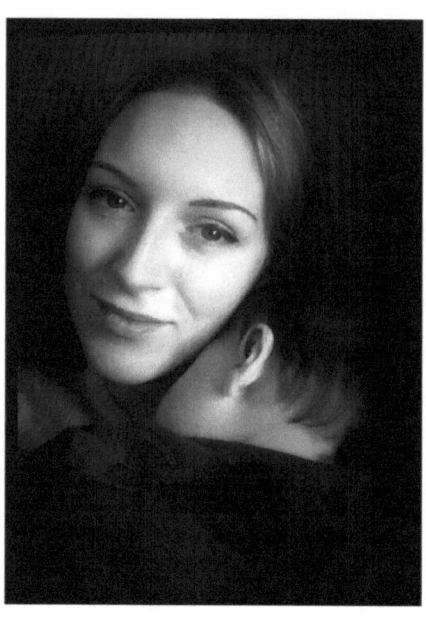

So my first step was to make peace with my appearance, which for the first 20yrs of my life I was entirely incapable of doing, but becoming a parent changed my perspective and made me see the world in a whole new light. I went from obsessing over my looks as a model to totally ignoring myself as a young parent. I took the bull by the horns one morning, stood naked in the mirror and cried my eyes out for how horrible my body looked; but it was ok to cry, I needed to, I needed to rid myself of the hurt and poison that I held inside of me, the cruel words of the bullies who had terrorised me for years and made me question my worth as a person. No matter what happened to me from that moment on the only way was up, I was willing and able to do anything that it took to regain my body, take control of my health for the right reasons this time and to be the healthy active mother that my daughter deserved. Stretch marks, saggy tits, flat arse, cat-bum stomach and thunder thighs will not defeat me, I'm more than just skin and flip-flops, I'm me and I deserve so much better. True beauty comes from within, it's deep within your bones, heart and soul, a kind personality, a warm smile. It doesn't matter what size your start from or end up at, it's the way that you hold yourself and view the world. I didn't want to be slim again to be beautiful, because I never felt beautiful anyway, but I wanted to be the best version of me that I could be, stronger, fitter, healthier and more able in life and that's exactly what a fit lifestyle can achieve.

I want you to use your emotion, your sadness and anger and turn it into positive energy, use it to drive yourself forward, to stay motivated and take steps each day to improve your life. So right now we're going to begin and I'd like you to take a photo of yourself, full length in the mirror in your underwear. This is a picture just for you so don't panic or stress about how you look because nobody has to see it, but it will tell your story and one day soon you will be so proud of how far you have come. If you've been crying, haven't showered, have hairy arm pits or mismatching underwear it seriously doesn't matter, this is your benchmark, your starting point and day one of the rest of your life. You will look back at this very photo and be astonished by how different your life is, and the people who meet you will never believe that you are the same person. Sometimes we need a visual marker to realise how far we have come in life, you know when you look back in a family album and feel shocked at how young everybody was, or how tall a cousin has suddenly become in the last couple of years. Having a photo to compare your results to keeps you on track, as you may not feel very different day to day, but when you have something to compare yourself to then suddenly you realise you're far slimmer, standing taller and looking healthier, and taking weekly pictures after giving birth really helped me to see that and keep me on track for another seven days of healthy living until I took my next progress picture. From as soon as I decided to change myself I made my pictures public to the world on my blog www.tracykiss.com because I knew then that I couldn't back out of it or give up. Not only did I not want to fail myself but I also didn't want to fail in front of others and it was a great incentive for me to keep going.

I sympathise with parents looking to get fit and lose weight, I know you work hard, I know you're tired in the evening after a draining day behind a desk and running around after the kids. I also know that cooking a dinner in the evening takes every ounce of energy and enthusiasm that you have left when you just want to collapse on the sofa and relax for a moment before going to bed and starting all over again. I know that your feet burn from standing, your eyes ache from working and you can't even be bothered to undo your shoelaces when you clamber through the front door. It's ok, I get it, I've been there and I'm still there, only with two children now but I made it through and you can too. Whilst it doesn't ever get easier you will certainly get better at it so that it feels less of a struggle the more capable your body becomes.

I also sympathise with people who have stressful jobs, not enough hours in the day and constant demands and deadlines. Stressing over sitting in traffic jams, running for the train, taking your work home with you, studying, researching, planning and fretting. Work is never done is it? As soon as you clear your desk there's another mountain forming from within your inbox before the kettles even whistled first thing in the morning. It's one step forwards and two steps back, and even when you're home at the end of a long day you can't switch off, can't sleep, feel restless and are still mentally planning for tomorrow well into the early hours when you're desperate to sleep.

Then there's the lack of self-esteem and money to join a gym, because going to a gym alone takes guts right? Skinny people stare at you and immediately you feel like you don't belong in an alien environment. You don't know the first thing about fitness, muscles or where to begin and a personal trainer costs more than your phone bill each month so there's no way you can afford expert help as well as a membership, parking costs and all of the spare time needed. And that's before arranging a babysitter for children and making sure dinner and homework is out the way before bedtime with a family. In an ideal world, if you were a celebrity with a childminder and the luxury of free time then of course you could workout everyday, but real people can't do that right? Wrong, they totally can.

I am a single mother of two young children, I have no childcare during the week just half an afternoon every Sunday after lunch and then it's back to the school run first thing on Monday morning. Yet I workout up to six days a week from home at no cost to myself and more importantly without taking anything from the shoestring budget that we live on.

Time Since Birth	6 days
Prev Wks Weight	12 st 7 lbs
Current Weight	11 st 0 lbs
Change	-21 lbs

Before you can consider working out and losing weight you first have to get your lifestyle in order so let's look back at the 39p food example. In place of money see calories, as food feeds our hunger right? The average male requires around 2,500 (calories) a day, women 1,900kcal and toddlers 1,300kcal so we obviously want to eat as much food as possible to stave off hunger without going over our daily allowance. If we eat too few calories we lose weight but feel hungry, eat the right amount we maintain our weight and feel content, but if we eat too many we will gain weight and feel bloated and sick.

I know that we still haven't got to the exercise bit yet, but lets keep that for later and concentrate on just our food for now, sit tight because it's coming. A common misconception that I see in people trying to lose weight is the fact that they limit their calorie intake in order to drop excess pounds, which sounds like it should work right? Eat less food to lose weight, makes sense. And it can, if you have the willpower to accompany it that is, but very few do, as we wouldn't be fat if we already had willpower to start with. At this present moment I haven't felt hungry in almost eight years and I don't think that I would be able to cope with hunger pains again as an adult because I eat so often my stomach is rarely completely empty. Hunger is hard, you feel hollowed out, your stomach constantly churns, you get dizzy, weak, irritable, angry and have pounding headaches, I wouldn't wish it on anyone, let alone deliberately choose to put myself through it again. And day-to-day we may feel peckish when it comes to meal time, but that slight discomfort is certainly not to the extreme of hunger, we're accustomed to eating so often that our stomachs are rarely ever empty and we pile more and more food down our throats before the last bite has even had time to digest. When you deny your body food you face the battle of hunger, telling yourself that you can lose weight by not eating, or eating far less than you should for as long as you can last, and by the time the symptoms of hunger kick in the majority of people give up. Of everyone I have seen dieting, the vast majority lose a little weight rather quickly and then put it straight back on again when they return to their normal lifestyle, if not ending up a little heavier than before they first started because they've binge eaten afterwards. Our bodies need food to function, for our organs to work and the processes to take place properly, and without food they can't do this.

I watch in horror as people live on mouse sized portions of food, feeling weak and angry and then crack and go on a junk food binge to boost their sugar levels and answer their cravings, on a single track road straight to diabetesville. I tell them not to do it and how dangerous it is for their health but they have tunnel vision and want a quick fix, determined to look good for a wedding or before going on holiday, yet quick fixes will never last, if something is worth doing then it's worth doing properly and it doesn't have to be a punishment. And without question of a doubt I have gone on to watch them continue to yo-yo with their weight without saying *I told you so*, because people see a slim woman and automatically think that she has no problem with her weight, when in actual fact we've worked the hardest to get to where we are, and continue to do so. The amount of food on a plate does not equate visually to its calorie intake, one single 5g square of chocolate from a plain milk chocolate bar contains 27kcal, one row of 25g chocolate contains 132kcal, 2 rows of 50g chocolate contains 265kcal and a 250g bar of milk chocolate contains about 1,320kcal. That's not even a lot of chocolate as I used to eat a 500g share bar of milk chocolate fruit and nut in one sitting to myself without coming up for oxygen and that's almost an entire days calorie intake for a woman, which was my snack after dinner, eek!

So let's look at what we can eat healthily for the same amount of calories. Our one square of chocolate for 27kcal can be replaced with a cup full of asparagus for 27kcal which would cover an entire dinner plate. I like to chargrill mine in a hot pan to keep it fresh and crisp but steaming it makes it sweet and succulent and it's a great detoxifying vegetable packed with vitamins, minerals and amino acids to help you to go to the toilet regularly and flush out excess fluids and toxins. I serve my asparagus hot on a bed of salad leaves with black pepper and it's out of this world, filling me up far more than one tiny cube of chocolate.

A row of chocolate comes in at 132kcal and takes all of two seconds to eat, for the same amount of 132kcal you can have a whole bowl of plain homemade popcorn that is wonderful for snacking. Not only does popcorn taste like it should be naughty but it also takes more time to eat than a row of chocolate, keeping your mouth busy for longer so you're less likely to go back to the snack cupboard for something else. Two rows of chocolate equates to 265kcal and for that you can have a 3oz sirloin steak, eggs and tomatoes, so my 500g bar of chocolate for 1,320kcal that I can embarrassingly finish before the end of an episode of Eastenders can literally provide me with an entire days worth of food. Let's try thirteen 100kcal meals to make up the equivalent calories shall we? For the same calories as a 500g bar of chocolate you can have a wholegrain crisp bread with cheese and tomato, a hot chocolate with marshmallows, a fruit salad, cheese and pickle on biscuits, strawberries and cream, smoked salmon and cream cheese, apples and peanut butter, baked beans on toast, a banana milkshake, a bowl of popcorn, a jacket potato, bowl of soup and granola, I don't think my stomach could physically hold that volume of food in one sitting and it's also far healthier in comparison.

But we all clearly like food or we wouldn't have eaten so much of it to have gotten to the size that we are, so denying ourselves the things that we love most will only make us crave them all the more, and we already know that we have no willpower to fight cravings, just as we dislike the pain of hunger. Healthy food is nowhere near as fun or enticing as naughty junk food, as it's packed with sugar and flavourings to purposefully keep us coming back for more, just like drugs, tobacco and alcohol. So how do we overcome stubborn cravings?

I seem to have an inbuilt safety switch installed by my cravings so that every time I tell myself that I won't eat any chocolate it suddenly becomes the only thing on my mind. My taste buds water with anticipation and my head fills with thoughts of biting down into chilled creamy blocks of cocoa heaven and after several minutes of fighting my urges I finally give in and go for a bite, telling myself that instead of having the entire bar I'll just have one square. But that one square tastes so good that within minutes I'm back for a second square and then a third, fourth and before I know it I've ate the entire bar. I always start off with good intentions to leave it well alone but unwittingly ended up eating it all and feeling guilty for breaking my rules. And because I feel guilty I tell myself that the day is a complete write-off and I'll start a fresh again tomorrow. As the sugar courses through my body I crave even more of it, so I go back to the snack cupboard to see if there's anything small perhaps that I can nibble on, and before I know it I've eaten cookies, biscuits, ice cream and honey coated nuts too and the vicious circle continues day after day with the *healthier tomorrow* never happening.

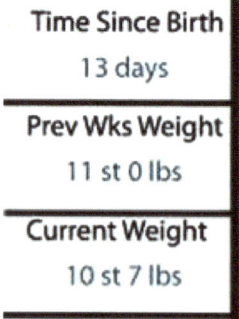

Time Since Birth
13 days
Prev Wks Weight
11 st 0 lbs
Current Weight
10 st 7 lbs
Change
-7 lbs

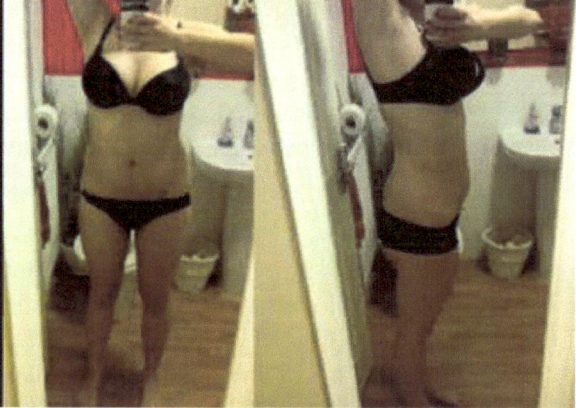

The only sure fire way to break the cycle of pigging out on junk food is to not buy any in the first place because if you don't keep snacks in the house then you can't eat them or feel guilty for failing yourself. Don't put yourself in a position to fall victim to your cravings, make a shopping list of healthy food items that you need to prepare your meals each week and only buy the things that you have written down. Don't let cheap deals lure you into stocking up on 2-for-1 snacks and reduced fat treats, you don't need it and it won't make you happy in the long run. A quick fix is only ever that. You only have to be strong for as long as it takes you to push a trolley around the supermarket, so make sure you do your weekly food shop straight after you've eaten a meal and that way you won't feel hungry or want to nibble as you shop so you'll be far less impulsive. When you get home if your cravings kick in then there'll be nothing in the house but healthy clean food which you can eat until your hearts content and after the first few days and weeks your body will have become accustomed to eating clean and no longer crave sugar.

The next step in sorting out your lifestyle is to replace junk food and convenience foods with conveniently healthy food. I can guarantee the majority of people who feel overweight and unhappy have either frozen chips, chicken nuggets, baked beans or pizza in their kitchen, if not all of them. Processed microwave or pre-packed oven meals will never be as healthy as a home cooked meal, and if you're serious about losing weight then you have to put in a little extra effort to tidy up your diet. Yes, cooking an entire meal from scratch after you've finished work is both tiresome and tedious, but if you cook enough for several meals at a time then you've got enough dinners, lunches or breakfasts to last an entire week, just increase your quantities for the amount you need and pop the rest into the fridge or freezer. Preparing homemade meals in advance of when they're needed, or meal prepping, is the perfect way to take control of meal times and each week I make up a giant cooking pot of brown rice, broccoli, cumin seeds, garlic, mushrooms and carrots with a vegetable stock cube and a splash of dark soya sauce and spoon it into plastic tubs to keep for a hot and healthy calorie conscious breakfast or lunch throughout the week, as without it I'd be pushed for time in the morning doing the children's breakfast and lunches that I'd probably end up eating toast or cereal for quickness which is loaded with carbs and sugar. If you bulk cook five different dinners one week then you'll have a months worth of meals for the family and three weeks off of cooking, just make sure you have enough space to chill or freeze them properly. I also make up homemade soups from sticks of celery and left over broccoli stalks usually with lentils or chickpeas, and that way no food is ever wasted because I cook up whatever is left over in the fridge or cupboard before doing my weekly shop each week; love food, hate waste!

And whilst we're on the topic of soups I'd just like to expose my biggest annoyance towards yo-yo dieters, as for some inexplicable reason people seem to think that blending up soup into nothing more than coloured water will make you skinny if you consume liquid meals day and night. Whilst it will certainly make your toilet times disgustingly messy, the moment you go back to solid food you'll put the weight straight back on again, you are not a baby, if you can eat a meal through a straw then it's not a meal. Watery soups are never satisfying enough to fill you up no matter how much you have, your body will always crave something solid after. Don't get me wrong, soups are delicious and I highly recommend you have them as part of a healthy lifestyle, but you must always make your own to ensure they are healthy and if you absolutely have to blend them then only blend or mash half of the ingredients and leave the other half hand chopped, this way the soup will be thick instead of watery and have enough texture to it for you to chew and feel as though you've actually had a meal.

My rule of thumb for meals is to make everything from scratch and if it comes premade then it's not for me. Wherever possible try to avoid packet mixes, sauces, toppings and instant food. If a factory can make it to survive several years in the back of a dark cupboard then you're capable of making a single fresh alternative at home. Ditch calorific salad dressings for extra virgin olive oil with salt and pepper for seasoning, switch ketchup on greasy fish and chips for baked salmon with juicy vine tomatoes and jacket potatoes and trade pasta and spaghetti for cous cous or pearl barley. Every meal that you can buy premade you can make a homemade healthier, lower calorie alternative and it will taste far nicer whilst keeping your cravings at bay because it won't be loaded with sugars, fats and preservatives to keep your body hooked on junk.

Perhaps the biggest change you can make immediately to your lifestyle is to monitor what you drink, as liquid may seem to slip under the calorie radar as it's not a food and doesn't fill you up, but it can be just as bad as bingeing on sweets and crisps when trying to lose weight because drinks are absolutely loaded with empty calories containing no nutritional value at all. I only drink water or green tea, and from hating liquid as a child I have now accustomed myself to drink several glasses of water a day that I have built up gradually as my tolerance to feeling floaty adjusts itself. I started off with sipping a small bottle of water throughout an entire day to keep a check of my intake, then I introduced a cup of green tea with my lunch, then another cup with breakfast and dinner and finally a small glass of water every couple of hours throughout the day, not only does it keep my body hydrated but it also flushes out the toxins and my urine has changed from dark to clear indicating I have consumed enough fluid. So let's take a look at the empty calories in traditional drink choices and the amount that they can add up to in an average day. A glass of pure fruit juice such as apple, orange or pineapple has around 110kcal, the same as a slice of toast. A can of Coca-Cola has 142kcal the same as a chocolate pudding, and a cup of white tea or coffee around 80kcal with a latte coming in at 110kcal which is the same as a few mouthfuls of chocolate.

On average tea and coffee drinkers have around 4-8 cups a day which can amount to around 640kcal extra calories or the equivalent of eating a second dinner every evening, now that's pretty scary for nothing more than liquid! Switching hot drinks for a cup of green tea is not only calorie free but it also great for your health with antioxidants and nutrients to improve brain function and dental health, assisting in fat loss and lowering the risk of cardiovascular disease, cancer and type II diabetes. Just switching your cool drinks for water or hot drinks for green tea each day is the equivalent of using a skipping rope for a straight hour at a constant pace, and seeing as I can hardly puff and pant my way past a few minutes of jiggling about and getting all sweaty whilst tangling my legs up, I can shave off those calories without having to lift a finger, I just boil the kettle.

It's all about being calorie wise and making little changes each day to amount to a large difference consistently over time. That 640kcal daily saving in tea amounts to 4,480 calories a week, 17,920 calories a month and 215,040 calories a year, making a whopping 61lbs in weight or 4st that you can save yourself each year without having to do any exercise at all. Now take that notion and apply it to other aspects of your diet. Instead of taking sandwiches everyday for lunch try bringing in a homemade soup once or twice a week, change sugary cereals for porridge oats with fresh fruit, stock the snack cupboard with rice cakes, unsalted nuts and dried fruits instead of biscuits, crisps and chocolate, and ditch packet bought puddings for oven baked bananas or homemade fruit smoothies.

The best advice that I can give to people about food is to enjoy it for it's freshness, taste and texture, make time to sit down at a table when eating each meal, chew every mouthful properly and savour the experience instead of rushing or talking while you eat. Use fresh quality ingredients to prepare home cooked meals that you love, because no amount of chewing on salad leaves will ever quench the appetite of a hungry carnivore. You have to eat until you feel full, until you're satisfied and then there will be no risk of snacking after dinner. Don't stuff yourself senseless, but equally don't starve yourself either, think about a healthy amount and remain consistent with your portion sizes. There's no point in living on grass if you follow it up with a tub of ice cream or bar of chocolate. You do not need to have a dessert every day; sugar is not compulsory. A treat is best enjoyed as a treat, not a part of your daily routine, so think more along the lines of once a week or even once in a blue moon and that way you'll enjoy it far more. The longer you go without eating junk food the less it will appeal to you, and eventually you won't want it at all because your body will feel far better eating healthy clean food that fills you with energy and keeps your system functioning as it should. One day you'll look at greasy stodgy bland or sickly sweet food and wonder what you ever saw in it, just like a cheating ex-boyfriend.

So after having my daughter I began making these changes and I gradually pulled my chaotic days into some sort of a routine, tightening and tweaking it as I went. When I made up her potato, carrot or apple purees I put an extra pot of vegetables on for myself. I bulk cooked my dinner to be able to meal prep for the week ahead and I made sure that I always sat down to eat breakfast, lunch and dinner with at least one glass of water to accompany every meal. Despite not being able to exercise for six weeks after birth I found that changing the way that I handled my food made such an incredible difference to my body, and as I got my newborn into a routine of eating and sleeping I also found my own routine of eating and sleeping too. I caught little naps throughout the day and night when she would sleep for an hour or two at a time. I made sure I ate my healthy vegetarian meals to keep my energy levels constant and dropped the junk food and empty calories and my body responded amazingly without ever having to step foot in the gym.

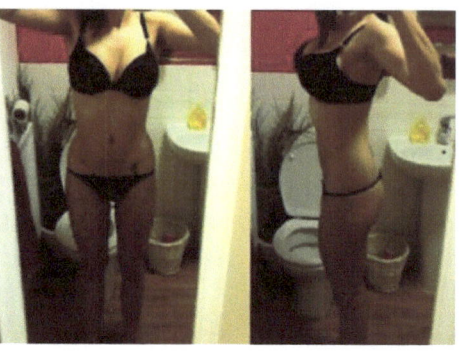

Time Since Birth	266 days
Prev Wks Weight	8 st 7 lbs
Current Weight	8st 7lbs
Change	-0lb

You don't have to be vegetarian or vegan to be skinny or lose weight because calories comes in all different shapes and sizes as I have shown you. I became a vegetarian as a child because I disliked the taste of meat and loved animals, and now as an adult I have converted to veganism, removing all dairy products from my diet and I have never felt better. I'm not here to preach to you about what you should and shouldn't be eating to be slim, but I'm just telling you what worked for me. And as 80% of what size you are equates to the food that you put into your mouth then other 20% of your physical activity seems pretty miniscule in comparison. There's no point in working out at the gym seven days a week for hours on end and destroying yourself if you're still drinking several cups of coffee a day, because you won't even break even on calories let alone lose weight, you'll just feel rubbish for putting in so much physical effort for zero results. So clean up your diet and then think about getting fit.

I'm not saying that you can't drink a milkshake ever again or eat Frosties for breakfast, but just try to have everything in moderation, instead of eating not-so-healthy foods everyday make it every other day, switch one day a week for a healthy eating day and then gradually increase it until it becomes everyday. Making a lifestyle change isn't about shocking your system and punishing yourself, it's all about making small changes over a period of time to one day reach your desired goal. Your goal should be to get fit and healthy forever, not just for a week whilst sitting on the toilet squeezing your insides out and having headaches from hunger pains before you cave in and go back to being reckless with junk food again. Nobody has time to be a yo-yo dieter!

So now that we've tackled the big bad wolf that is our diet we can finally start to look at exercise. And for some, just the mention of exercise is enough to send the majority of us running for the sofa to go and put our feet up. Life is tough, I get tired easily and I have hardly any time to sit down and relax with my children let alone jump about in spandex. But the best form of exercise is the kind that doesn't actually feel like exercise, the stuff that takes next to no effort but makes a great difference, and something that we can sneak into our daily routine to constantly knock off those calories day by day, one pound at a time.

One of my biggest tips for getting in shape is to ditch transport and use your feet, and a great example of this is the school run. I live about a mile, or a twenty-minute walk from school and have to drop the children to the school gates every morning for 9am. I collect my son from preschool at 12am and my daughter again at 3pm walking there and back each time which amounts to six twenty-minute walks each day, or three return trips totalling two hours of gradual constant exercise burning around 280kcals each day and 1,400kcal each school week which is over a days worth of calories!

When my son was first born I used to drive to school because I thought that it would be easier than taking him in a pushchair, carrying nappy bags and trying to get along the congested footpaths on four wheels outside the school gates; but in actual fact it's far more stressful driving as I have to queue along the entire road in traffic, struggle to find a parking space amongst the houses, curbing my wheels parallel parking on a congested road and getting held up by pedestrians crossing to get to school. After all that I still have to get the children out of the car, bags on backs, lock up and walk into school which can be several minutes away depending on where I eventually get parked, and the whole fiasco takes about the same amount of time as walking when you consider waiting in traffic and getting parked. Add to the equation the cost of driving being about £0.15p per mile, then my six miles a day in the car costs me £0.90p or £4.50 each week, £18.00 a month and £216.00 a year, for that we could have a few family days out, picnics and toys simply for leaving the car on the drive.

Not only does walking to and from school save on the stress and hassle of traffic jams and parking at peak time, but it also gives us the chance to talk about our day, enjoying some quality family time and looking at pretty flowers, animals and views that we pass en route. We frequently play I-spy and counting games to help my little ones with numbers, shapes, colours and sums as we pass by house numbers, post-boxes and road signs. I often ask them to look for a certain animal or type of architecture which improves their concentration, spatial awareness and memory.

And if you don't have children to worry about the morning school run then consider reducing the car journeys that you take on a daily or weekly basis; perhaps park a little further way from work and walk half the distance, instead of taking the bus from home walk to the next stop and then get on, or buy a bike and cycle if there are safe cycle routes to where you are heading. If you're a stay at home parent then the school run is a great way to get consistent daily exercise and the children will be far healthier for it, having a better appetite for dinner and sleeping more soundly at night for being active.

For some reason we seem to think that we have very little free time during the day, when in actual fact we have bags of it but choose to fill it with unnecessary actions that neither challenge nor motivate us. Take for example the average person working five days a week between the hours of 9am-5pm. Let's say they spend an hour a day travelling to and from work which totals nine hours of being away from home. Let's also say that they go to bed at 10pm each evening and wake up at 7am giving them nine incredible hours of sleep, which I would just like to mention that I've hardly seen more than six hours a night in the past several years. So work and sleep totals eighteen hours for the average person, as there are twenty-four hours in a day this leaves six hours spare, so we'll be generous and allocate three of those hours to having breakfast, lunch and dinner, although lunch is also included in a working day, yet this still leaves three hours spare each day after all work, travel and generously allocated meal times are done and dusted. Of these three hours surely you can spend an hour, half an hour or even ten minutes a day being active, and at a weekend let's presume the average person has one day off of work which leaves twelve whole hours spare, that's half an entire day!

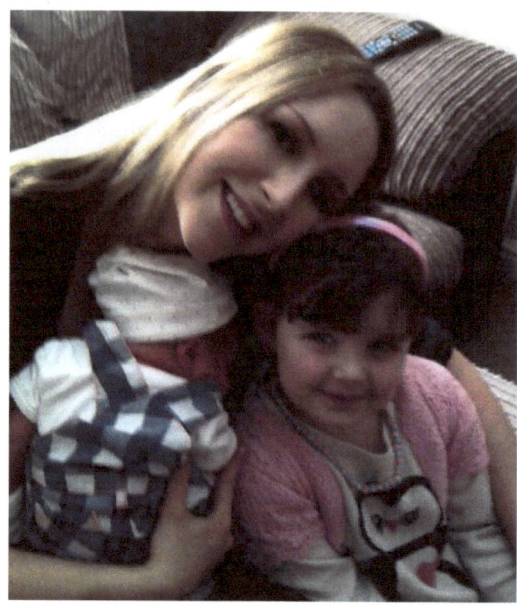

I also know that people love to watch television, which is something that I no longer have the luxury of since having children as I use my spare time to tidy up, do the dishes, laundry, meals and help with their homework before bath time, bedtime and a little bit of sleep before the morning routine starts all over again. Yet with the nation hooked on soaps, sitcoms and satellite television it's become the norm for people to come home from school and work and spend the entire afternoon and evening sitting on the sofa to watch episodes and entire series on a daily basis. Now my advice is switch it off and enjoy your family, go to the park or play in the garden, but for those who love the escapism of television I'm not here to tell you that you can't have it anymore, but instead use it to your advantage.

Let's say the average duration of a daily soap opera is thirty minutes at a time, split into two fifteen minute sections with a couple of minute ad break in between. So how about each time your favourite soap comes on TV you use it as your cue to call to do some exercise. Start off by placing a foot stool on the floor in front of you and when it gets to the ad break stand up and step on an off of it at a steady pace until the program comes back on again. As you get comfortable with this why not try to step for the first fifteen-minute section of the program and eventually the whole half an hour. Take it slow, take it at your own pace and realise that every step you take is one more than you would have taken if you'd sat on the sofa the entire time. You still get to watch your soap opera, you still have the exact same amount of spare time left over in your day but you've just completed a workout and burned around 290kcal whilst being distracted by the television, so you hardly notice the gentle exercise you're taking but you get the result of losing weight and toning up. Do it every day, keep it up and increase your pace and steps taken and before you know it you'll be a few dress sizes down without huffing and puffing in a gym or feeling sick.

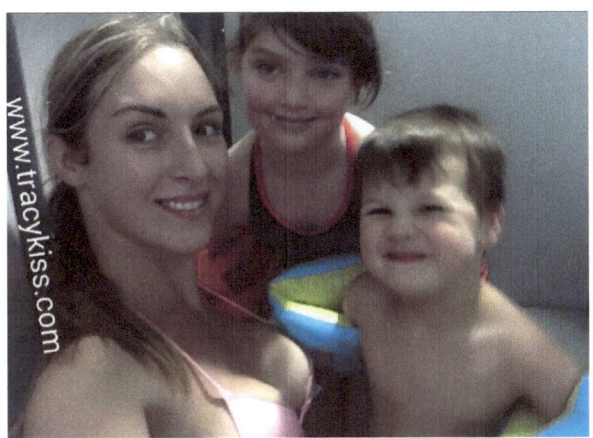

If you want to take your indoor exercise to the next level try getting some ankle weights which are adjustable weighted cuffs that velcro around your legs, making your muscles work a little harder to step up and down and in turn burning more calories for the same amount of movement. Get yourself some dumbbells to hold whilst stepping and move your arms alternately back and forth at the same pace and you have a whole body workout that not only burns fat but also tones and tightens every inch of you. If you don't have dumbbells then hold a tin of baked beans or a bottle of water and you can sip it as you go.

I find pedometers are great for making you aware of how active you are during the day, as they're a small electronic device that you attach to your clothing or wrist and track your movement to record how many steps you take. I have a FitBit which is a wristband that links to an app on my iphone and tracks my sleep pattern to tell me my optimum time to rest, it also monitors my level of activity throughout the day and informs me of how many more steps or exercise that I need to take to reach my daily goal, and it even charts and calculates the calories in my meals so that I know how much I can eat or drink to stay within my daily allowance. To build a healthy lifestyle you have to remain consistent and make small gradual changes to your attitude and activity, the results won't be as fast as a crash diet or extreme fitness program, but once the foundations are in place the changes will take effect and last a lifetime without your weight ever yo-yoing which is priceless. I find tracking progress in stats and figures is particularly rewarding for my OCD as you can compare steps week by week, monitor calories burned and predict how long it will take to shed the excess pounds based over a period of time and activity; a far healthier way to take control of your body than trying to starve yourself or survive on soup alone.

If you feel that you're ready to actually go for a full on workout then I'm a massive fan of Beachbody USA who produce home workout DVD's that you can do from the comfort of your lounge, bedroom, hotel room or staffroom with little or no equipment necessary. They contain full workout programs, meal plans and step-by-step personal instructors performing each workout with people of all ages and abilities joining in and modifying moves so that you don't have to feel left behind or incapable. The stronger you get and the more supple you become the harder you can make each move in your own time by adding weights or going deeper into stretches, lunges or squats; there is always a modified, easy and hard version of each exercise available. And there's a whole host of workouts to choose from depending on what kind of exercise you're looking to do. For the more meaty and extreme sweat-inducing workouts then Insanity and Insanity Max: 30 are pretty awesome, for those short of time Focus T25 is a concise daily burst of exercise, and for something a little more relaxed then PiYo is a wonderful fusion of Pilates and yoga, with dance routines and weight intensive plans too. I've stocked up on inexpensive home gym equipment over the years with a few dumbbells, ankle weights, resistance bands and a pull up bar as my staple pieces, along with yoga mats and a vertical pole for pole fitness, and it all pops away into a sports bag to store in my cupboard until needed whilst taking up very little space.

Being fit and healthy involves handling life in moderation, take everything one step at a time, know your limits and gradually try to extend them when you feel confident and able to, there's no need to rush or burn yourself out. Start by straightening out your mind, removing the stresses from your daily life and dealing with the reason why you are the size you are. Being fat isn't ugly, there is no size to determine beauty but you deserve to be happy in yourself and to feel good, and generally the better your health inside the better you feel about yourself on the outside. Quit smoking, stop taking drugs and switch alcohol for water, then look at decreasing and eliminating junk food entirely from your daily routine. If you can make the leap to vegetarianism or even veganism then you'll notice the biggest difference in your energy levels and health, but don't panic if you can't give up meat and dairy, just be calorie wise and seek healthy alternatives whenever possible.

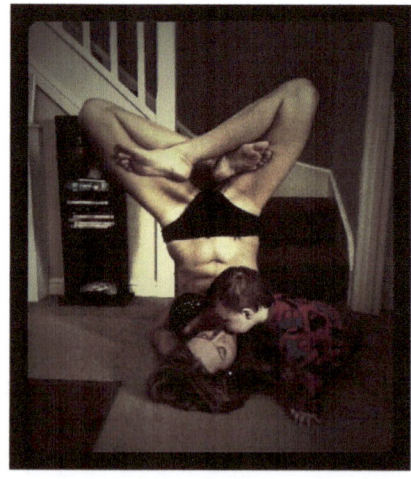

Don't punish yourself and don't give yourself a hard time if and when you mess up, we're all human, we all have our good days and bad. Just go at life with a positive mind, say yes to new challenges and never be afraid to broaden you horizon. Recognise when you're being greedy or lazy and take steps away from that kind of behaviour, because every step that you take brings you one closer to your goal. People are often amazed at how calm and controlled I am in the face of chaos, how I run a household, family and work around my two children as a single parent whilst being in the best shape of my life, always smiling and inspiring others to do the same. I'm not a celebrity, I'm not on drugs and I don't have a team of staff, childminders and cleaners to do it all for me; I'm just a normal girl leading a normal life that I decided to take charge of. I split everything into what is necessary and what is unnecessary, I watch what I spend so that I never get into debt, I put thought into the food that I buy to ensure my children are healthy and energetic, and I manage my time by minimising laziness and building a strong and reliable routine which gets easier and more efficient each time that I go through it.

Gone are the days of being a care free, starving hungry, sickly skinny and moody teenager and now I'm a positively beaming and proud parent with the body of my dreams and a zest for life and I hope that my words will help to transform you on the same journey that I have taken. Believe in yourself and you will achieve greatness, start your transformation today and stop making excuses. Little and often is the best way to introduce change to your life and each step that you take brings you one closer to reaching your goal. Your happiness is key; longevity brings success, and each day you will become that little bit stronger, more confident and able to continue along the right path at a pace that you set and are comfortable with.

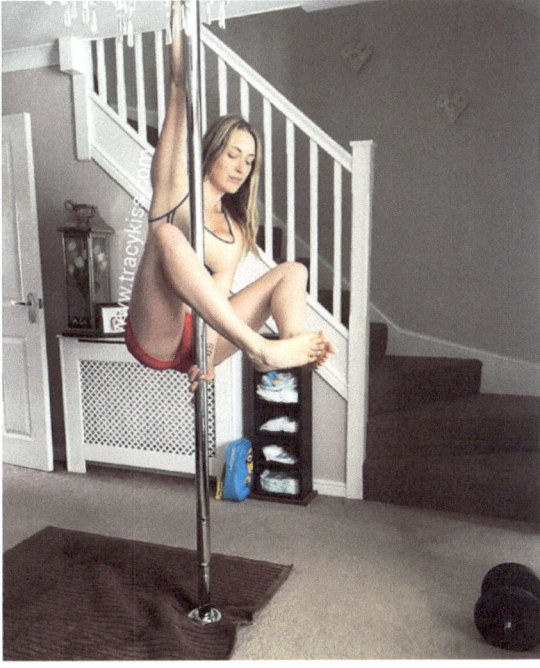

It's vital that you keep a positive can-do attitude and if you start saying *yes* to things it will have the most amazing influence on your mindset and activity rate. For example, whenever I sit down I immediately hear the words "Mummy can I have…?" as my children see that I am idle and magically feel thirsty, hungry or want a toy from some far off shelf in the bedroom. Instead of saying "In a minute" I immediately say "yes" and I get up and do it without hesitation. If I were to ask them to wait the issue will still be there in another several minutes only they'll probably become anxious or more desperate for me to do it, which in turn builds stress and annoyance. Simply getting up and doing it straight away takes the action off of my to-do list and keeps my little ones happy without anyone becoming agitated. Likewise, when I'm on my way to retrieve what they've asked for I'm also getting exercise, and as I pass things along the way I pick up a dirty cup and carry it with me into the kitchen which leads to my house getting tidier. On the way upstairs I sometimes take some toys back up with me to return them to the children's toy box, and on the way back downstairs I bring the bathroom bin down to empty it. Incorporating these little tasks into the actions you are already doing will help you to stay on top of housework and speed up the time you spend cleaning, as you tag it into your daily activity.

My house is absolutely spotless, immaculately tidy and always like a show home as I am very house-proud and dislike mess and chaos. I like everything to have a place and everything to be necessary. Clutter will only stress you out; it makes it harder for you to find the things that you needs, provides distractions from what you are doing and takes far more effort to tidy away a mess at the end of the day than doing it bit by bit as you make it. I recommend spending a weekend going through each room, recycling or selling old, unused or broken things and having a good clearout; a clean and tidy home allows for a clean and tidy mind. I never have mountains of washing, I don't ever leave dirty dishes in the sink and my children know whatever toys they get out have to get put away before they can play with another one or go to bed. Not only does this keep our home clean and tidy at all times but it also teaches my children to look after their belongings, to treat them with respect and help out with chores such as feeding the animals or unloading the washing machine. And of course they're children and I don't limit their fun; they're free to jump and climb, paint and role play wherever and however they choose, but every night before bed I make sure the house is spotless so that when we wake up in the morning all we have to do is get on with the day ahead rather than cleaning up the mess from yesterday. It's all too easy to roll over mess and chores to tomorrow and the next day by always saying "I'll do it later" and before you know it you have an avalanche on your hands that's impossible to control.

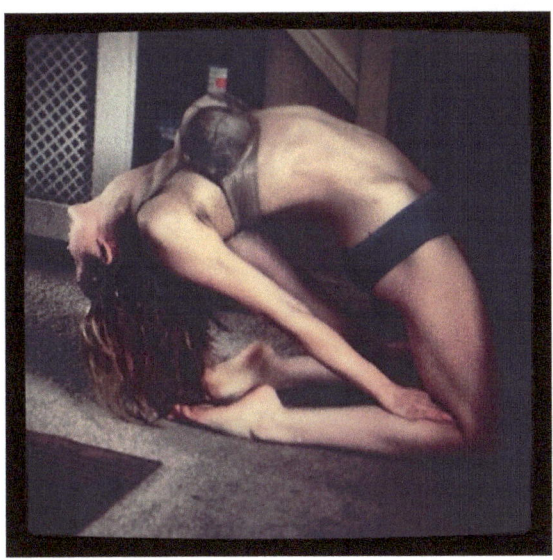

If you find the morning routine a panic and mad rush to get yourself or everyone else washed, fed, dressed and out of the door on time then shift your day back half an hour or so. Instead of getting up at 07:30am get up at 07:00am instead and go to bed half an hour earlier. You still get the same amount of sleep, you still have the same amount of free time during your day but you've just simplified your deadline for being out of the door by giving yourself longer to complete your daily routine. Rather than rushing and panicking as you jump out of bed, wake up and stretch, take your time to visit the bathroom and empty your bowels, shower and eat a nutritional breakfast to give yourself the energy to start your day, never skip breakfast because it's the most important meal of the day. When you feel good and look after yourself you will have more energy, a better outlook on life and positive attitude that overflows into everything that you do. If getting to work during rush hour stresses you out then consider asking your boss if you can start your shift an hour earlier and finish an hour earlier at home time; moving your day back slightly will allow you to skip the morning and evening traffic jams and still allow you a full day at work whilst possibly cutting your travel time in half. If you start your morning tired, stressed out and flustered then your entire day will be a write off because of it, do not let stress beat you because it will only make you fail and feel less capable. Take a deep breath, close your eyes and compose yourself, you are in control.

Look over your day and make a list of which issues and activities test you; the school run, getting to and from work, making dinner, doing the housework, walking the dog even, and see how better you can manage your time. You could walk the dog to and from school with you instead of driving, meal prep your dinners so that you're only cooking three times a week instead of seven, delegate some tidying or cleaning chores to the children to earn their pocket money and ask your partner to help out more around the house. Throw away your washing up tub in the kitchen sink so that at meal times you always have to wash your pots and pans up before you sit down to eat; this way the food doesn't dry out and get stuck on so it's twice as fast and easy to clean off rather than leaving it for later when you have to soak and scrub at it. Rinse your plates and cutlery straight after you eat and put them away and the kitchen will always remain beautifully clean and hygienic.

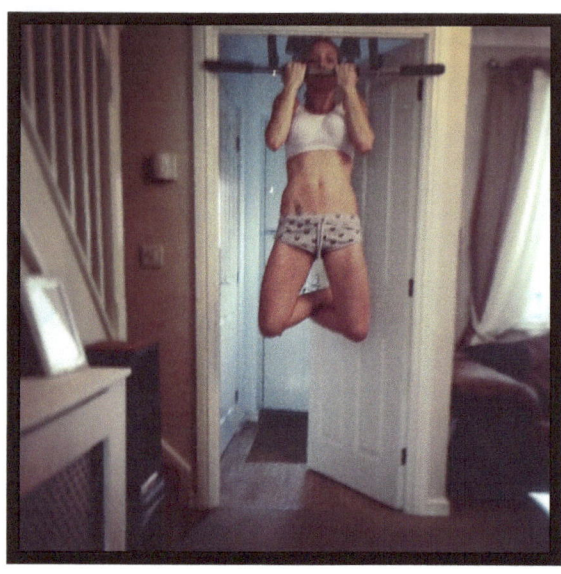

If you stick to the same routines each day and manage your time effectively you will fall into an effortless pattern to optimise your activities. All too often I see families with messy dirty houses, broken toys and piles of washing and clutter everywhere. Once you've got your home clean and tidy it's far easier to keep it that way, and when you go to bed at night with a pristine house you won't lay awake worrying about all of the things that need to be done in the morning. If a light bulb blows then change it, if a handle breaks replace it, it's far easier to sort something out as soon as it happens than to leave it broken and have to work around it, unable to close a door, see in a dark room or use kitchen equipment; it will only ever lead to wasting your time, making your life harder or stashing away more mess for you to tackle later. If it's broken throw it away, if you need it then fix or replace it. You wouldn't get on an aeroplane with one wheel or a broken wing, so don't live in a home that's unsafe and untidy. When everything is in order you'll never lose your keys, never fall behind on chore and never panic when the doorbell rings and unexpected guests arrive.

I fell pregnant with my son at the age of twenty-five when my fiancé decided the time was right to try for a baby. This time around my outlook and lifestyle was far healthier than when I was a teenager and in just a few years I'd become a domestic Goddess. I proudly walked my daughter to school with my blooming baby bump before driving off to work for the day and being home in time to cook the dinner. I ate healthily, worked right up until I gave birth and had a very speedy natural delivery and a healthy baby boy to bring home to meet his big sister. Again I put on a lot of pregnancy weight, not quite as much as the first time around but I still had a great appetite and ate larger portions even though they say you shouldn't eat for two! I realised my love for food and replaced the snacking of my first pregnancy with hearty homemade meals of larger portions and plenty of fruit and green leafy vegetables. My second pregnancy was a bit of a treat time for me in the sense that I didn't have to limit my portion sizes quite so strictly, and for ten months I dabbled with second helpings of dinner and the occasional extra healthy snacks. I also tool a pregnancy supplement to ensure my son received all of the vitamins required to help him to grow properly without draining my own energy and reserves, which prevented me from fainting and being weak this time. For my second pregnancy I was as strong as an ox and felt so much more human because my body was properly nourished. My son was born at 39wks just like my daughter but a whopping 8lbs8oz, a whole 1lb 8oz heavier than my daughters birth weight with four and a half years between them.

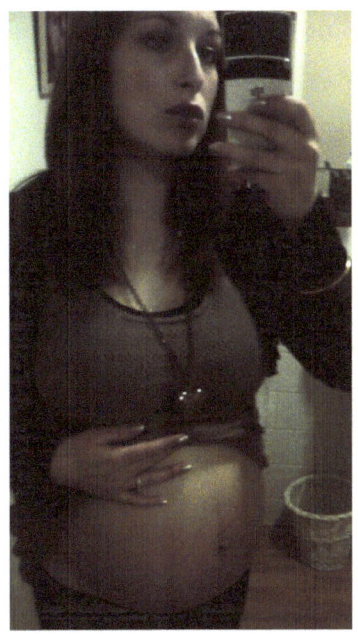

I took to being a mother of two in my stride, falling back into the routine of breastfeeding, sleepless nights, school runs and weaning, and this time if was far easier because I already knew how to do it all properly from the get go and wasn't unsure or doubtful of my actions. If my son cried I'd automatically pick him up and give him a kiss, sniff his nappy, wind him over my shoulder or put him to my breast which removed the hours of crying for no apparent reason, alleviated trapped wind quickly and left him comfortable and content with our home peaceful and happy. Like everything in life the more times you do it the better you get at it, and eventually it becomes second nature and isn't a chore at all. I love raising my children and I love taking care of my family and myself, we are all happy, healthy strong individuals who always smile and do our best at everything we undertake. You will never fail at anything in life so long as you never stop trying.

Unfortunately several months after my son was born my breast implants ruptured and the silicone leaked into me, it left me in severe pain as my chest collapsed and prohibited my circulation leaving me short of breath and very weak. I had to have my eight-year-old implants removed and breast reconstructive surgery across two operations that left me bed ridden and on strong painkillers in a drowsy haze of unconsciousness. Five days after I came out of hospital my fiancé of six years left me, stating that he couldn't be responsible for a family and wanted to be young, free and single. It broke my heart and I was helpless to do anything, but I let him go without saying a word because I knew that he'd be happier on his own rather than being forced to be somewhere where he was no longer happy. It was then that I realised how much I do in life; I single headedly carried a mountain of responsibility on my shoulders but never batted an eyelid. And when it came to me going into hospital and handing over the reins to my fiancé it scared the hell out of him and he left. I'd become so capable in life that nobody around me had to lift a finger, and being trapped in my bed, healing and in pain I cried my eyes out for not being able to hug my children or straighten the duvet and fluff the pillows.

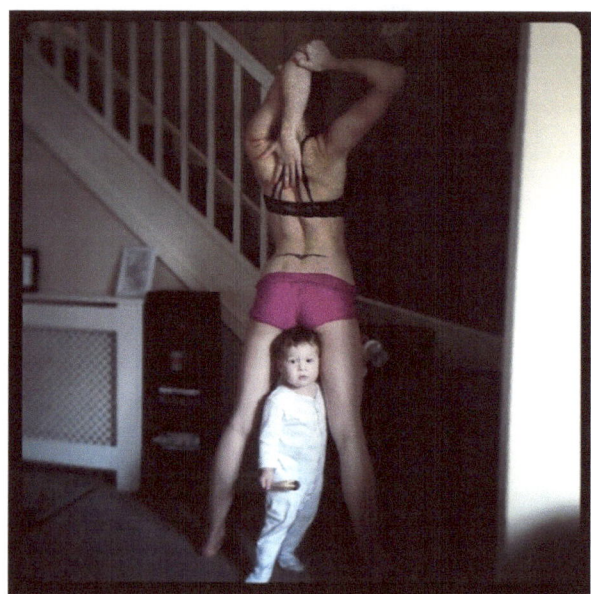

Day by day I became stronger as my body healed and I stopped taking my painkillers prematurely so that I could think straight and stay conscious. Despite my heart and body being broken I realised that I was at my lowest point in life and the only way was up. My surgeon checked me over and gave me the all clear to start lifting small things such as teacups and dinner plates but not yet raise my arms above my head because my body was still weak and needed to heal. I took his advice and regained my strength a little at a time as I gradually let go of the heartache and it gave me such freedom that I'd never felt before. Within a few months of having my reconstructive surgery I was back on track with my life, my two children happy and my body tight and toned and not an ounce of fat on me. I began bodybuilding, using dumbbells and weights, my pull-up bar and cycling on an exercise bike all from home around raising the children. I used my Beachbody programs to do yoga, Pilates, muscle programs and cardio to drop fat and build a strong core. My energy levels were through the roof, my home happy and tidy and my children seemingly unaffected by the breakup as they had their Mummy back to full health again. If anything, becoming a single parent made my life easier because I only have three people to look after now instead of four.

All too often people are ruled by fear in life and it stops them from achieving their dreams. Scared of being alone, scared of being rubbish at something, scared of what other people might think or say about them. Stop being scared, you get one life so live it for what makes you truly happy and give everything your best shot. Nobody is perfect, nobody starts off an expert the first time that they try something and we're all here to learn, grow and achieve as we go. In the past eight years I've gone from a selfish, moody teenager who starved herself to a strong and powerful single mother of two. My life is brimming with positivity, love and encouragement and I'm extremely humbled and proud to help hundreds of thousands of people worldwide to achieve the body of their dreams. I'm not a celebrity, I haven't been photo shopped and I don't live on blended baby food or diet of pills. I'm just an average girl who has two children and the body of her dreams and you can too.

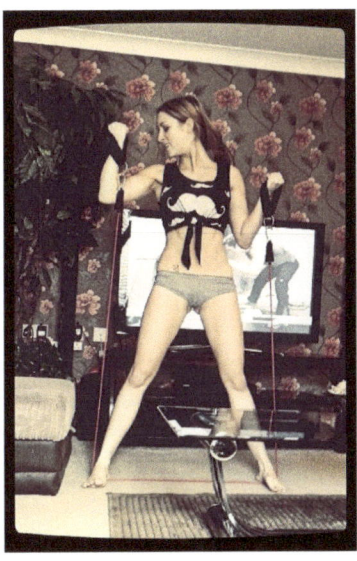

Remember your lifestyle is controlled by your mindset, start saying yes to everything and deal with your tasks and problems head on straight away; clear your mind, take control of your life and eat the foods that make you feel great inside instead of sluggish. Hydrate your body with water, cleanse your home and mind and keep active one baby step at a time. If you want to exercise then try some DVD workouts from home before building up to a gym membership if you have the spare time and money; and if you can't manage an hour of exercise in one go then break it up into three twenty minute sections after each meal throughout the day. Do everything in moderation, eat well, rest well and always put your health and wellbeing first. You can do this and you will do this, I have every faith in you and I look forward to seeing your before and after photos.

#teamkiss
www.tracykiss.com

www.ingramcontent.com/pod-product-compliance
Lightning Source LLC
Chambersburg PA
CBHW050758290526
45792CB00008B/2230